.

SITACISE©!

Just Sit and Get Fit!

Sitacise Just Sit and Get Fit!

By Mr. Mark D. & Kathy M. Brown, I.

Mark & Kathy Brown are certified master level and personal trainers respectively. They have been involved in fitness for over a combined 70 years. They have trained with Olympic gold medalist, pro football and basketball players, and world-class sprinters. They have created fitness programs, produced several fitness DVDs, have written fitness books, led and instructed many fitness programs and work with school systems youth creating, developing and implementing fitness programs.

The Sitacise© book, full-size movement chart, Movement DVDs and other products are available at www.Sitacise.com All product are produced, created and designed at MDB1 Studios© all rights reserved.

Mark and Kathy Brown can be contacted for seminars, speaking engagements and program development at mbrown1@neo.rr.com.

Always get a physical first before doing Sitacise movements and exercises. Do these movements & exercises at your own risk.

Exercises & movements are unique and personal and your personal results are dependent on your effort and performance. Always do the best that you can for yourself because you are special and very very important! You are worth the best you have to offer yourself! Take your time & get healthy and fit at your own pace.

SITACISE!

Join

The

SITACISE!

Movement

Now!

Just

Sit

And

Get

Fit!

Anywhere that you sit is a place to get fit!

SITACISE!

Sitacise©, just sit and get fit, anyplace you sit! Now comes a program that is going to allow you to get healthy and fit in any chair, on any couch, on any seat that you will sit! And you can do it without killing yourself or even breaking a sweat! Sit & get fit at work, at home watching TV, playing video games, while at school, while your driving. All you have to do is just sit down and get fit, just sit and get fit, Just Sit and Get Fit!

Anyplace That You Can Sit, is A Place you Can Get Fit!

ANYWHERE!

JOIN THE JUST SIT AND GET FIT SITACISE MOVEMENT NOW!

Contents

Chapter 1

Fat or Fit! Are We Insane?

"The classic definition of being insane is to do the same thing over and over again and to expect a different result".

This quote has been attributed either to Ben Franklin or Albert Einstein. Which ever one of these gentlemen made this quote really does not matter, what matters is that for years we have been trying to correct our health, physical fitness and excessive weight problems by doing the same things over and over and over again and expecting a different result.

Only to find out that we continue to lose this year's version of the *"battle of the bulge"* once again and we are left wondering why? The following examples are things that individuals have told us that they have experienced and tried and that we have witnessed being tried, only to have the same outcome! Failure to obtain great health and weight loss! Read on and see if any of this sounds familiar to you.

We try to put on that same old exercise clothing that we used to wear years ago that's now much to tight and small and now we are really committed to getting in shape! As if those old clothes have some magical powers that are going to turn back the hands of time and make our bodies the same as they were back then. We pull out the same old physical fitness equipment that we utilized when we were much younger and we expect to work out like crazy even though we are not quite as young as we used to be. Even though it's been a few, quite a few years since we have even moved much at all, we are ready! Come on Let's do this! **It Ain't**

No Stopping Us Now!

We never even considered the fact that our metabolism has changed quite a bit and that we do not metabolize blood sugars and blood fats as efficiently as we used to. Back then we could eat almost anything we wanted to and that youthful food-burning furnace we called our body could burn up calories at an amazing pace!

We just put it in and burned it up at hyper speed. It was as if we all had hollow legs or something! The food just seemed to disappear and 10 minutes later we were eating again! What was so great is that our waistlines always stayed the same. WOW! You ladies remember those 36-24-36 measurements don't you?

We also may have been working a more vigorous type of job which required us to move quite a bit more during the day and burn more calories performing those tasks on our job back then, that we are not burning today! This is a very important point to remember because we will be discussing this point in great depth later. There is a new and very interesting body of study called "Inactivity Physiology" that is going to change the way everyone thinks about physical fitness routines and exercise as a whole.

We pulled out that same old exercise routine that we use to use and now we're ready to go! We're really are going to get it done! Here we go, look out world nothing can stop us now, we are really going to do this, we have the willpower, the determination to bring it, to kick some butt, to do it now! Within minutes, hours or days we give out and we give up and our exercise and get healthy comeback has failed once again!

There was this one woman and I don't want to use the word old, because old is something that we tend to throw away or discard. Like that *old dress* or those *old pair of shoes* that I'm going to get rid of or throw away. We like to use the words mature or vintaged. Like *"the mature disquished woman always looks great at any age"*. Or the vintaged, well-preserved automobile is worth more 50 years later then it was when it was new! If an automobile can look good at over 50 why can't we look good over 50? <u>**You Are Not a Throw Away or a Discard so Stop Treating Yourself As One and Start Treating Yourself like the Special Someone That You Are! And Start Doing It Right Now! You Are Worth It!**</u>

This mature woman that had not exercised in quite some time and she had gained a considerable amount of weight (almost 70 pounds in 10 years) and now she was ready to begin an exercise program. She claimed that in the past she had always received many compliments about her looks and that made her feel good! She said that however; over the years the compliments started to decrease as her weight and waistline begin to increase, until finally they stopped altogether.

This mature woman said that at first it hurt her very badly when she went into her closet to try to put on some of the clothing that she often got compliments in that now she was unable to wear them because of the weight she had gained. She said that over time she had to buy bigger and bigger clothes until finally she was wearing baggy sweat pants and big tops. She hated getting dressed up for anything because nothing seemed to "fit right".

But then this lady said something that really made us feel extremely sorry for her; she said that after awhile I started to feel as if I were invisible; as if no one saw me anymore. I just began to accept the fact that I would be overweight and unhealthy for the rest of my life. And this mature woman was a very well educated college graduate that was secure in her career, married and has put all her children through college. But she still wanted to look and feel good, not for her children, not for her husband, but she wanted to do it for herself!

Whenever we encounter anyone that is well preserved or vintaged we always make a big fuss over them and you should see them blush and smile! They always say the compliments make them feel good and makes them feel special!

We say things to them like " you look great, have you lost weight? What have you been doing to remain looking so GOOD? Or the big one is "YOU LOOK JUST LIKE YOU DID YEARS AGO! YOU NEVER CHANGE"! They really light up and began to smile then and they are happy to share their secrets of looking good with us.

This mature woman was trying to exercise more but she was making the one mistake that most make, she is trying to do it with old technology & on her <u>own</u> and has become discouraged and quit. It is so very important to make sure that one receives personal instruction or follows the advice of knowledgeable sources. Don't entrust your health to amateurs, not even to yourself. Get advice from fitness experts !

If one does not know how to get into shape and look great, even though you may have done some things in the past that worked, this is a different time and a different you. You need to apply a different strategy to your exercise philosophy that is geared toward the new environment that we live in today. The old things have not worked! But lest we digress, let us proceed. We know you're busy.

Or we watch one of those infomercials that are geared to inspire us to think that we can get one of those types of bodies that the models have on those infomercials. In just eight weeks, or 60 or 90 days we can look like they do! All we have to do is buy that program and we will be ripped like they are! But no one ever told us that we had to work that hard! And no one ever told us that often times those models, even the real-life ones worked out a whole lot more than the recommended times that the infomercial said you had to!

One of the most unique features about those infomercials is that no one ever tells you about the strains, sprains, torn and injured muscles, tendons, ligaments and injured joints that you may experience from doing these high intensity, high impact kinds of activities. Also there is always a disclaimer in very small fine almost microscopic print that reads: *results may vary depending on your own circumstances and that the result you see may not be typical of the results you will get!*

The only reason that we are watching this infomercial is because we were channel surfing and we saw these scantily clothed models with tremendously toned abdominal muscles, chiseled, hard legs and arms and over all totally ripped bodies and we stopped to find out what they were advertising and if there was any way that we could look like that! Then the infomercial assured us that if we would commit to working out and eating as outlined in the infomercial that we would get those results too.

Then the infomercial went on to tell us that if we were not completely satisfied for any reason that we could return the product no questions asked, and get all our money back! Then you tell us in teeny tiny microscopic print that our results may vary, ddduuuuuhhhh! We do not want our results to vary, we want to look just like those people who are in the infomercial, and if possible maybe even a little bit better, not worse! How dare you try to tell us that our results may vary. That sounds like false advertising to me, how about you fellow readers?

I get so mad when I see statements like or hear statements like that! I feel like I'm been cheated and ripped off! I feel as if someone has been trying to trick or deceive me! How about you fellow readers? Do you feel cheated again?

We have just done the same old thing again, trying all of these crazy, nutty, difficult, just plain hard and sometimes insane physical fitness and exercise programs that have failed in the past and hoping that they will succeed for us today! What is wrong, what's the problem or problems and what can we do to solve them? It is a very obvious fact that we have not resolved the problem yet, individually or as a nation, America.

If we had resolved this problem, experts would not be predicting 75% of us Americans would become obese by 2015! Before we move on we cannot strongly reiterate that our health is much to important to put into the hands of amateurs, committees, friends that know a little about working out ect. Uncle Bob's a nice guy but would you have him give you a perm?

Would you have him work on your teeth? Your body and your health are much more important then those! Think about it! This is too important even for you to handle if you don't know what your doing! Get a great not good personal trainer or other qualified person for help!

Chapter 2

The Prediction and the Problem

It has been predicted by researchers Youfa Wang, Assistant Professor in the Department of International Health at the Johns Hopkins Bloomberg School of Public Health and May A. Beydoun, also from John Hopkins, that by the year 2015, 75% of all Americans adults will be overweight. Professor Wang also caution that "Obesity is a public health crisis and that nearly 24% of US children and adolescents will be overweight or obese." In a sobering final comment, the scientists warned that "Obesity is likely to continue to increase and if nothing is done, it will soon become the leading preventable cause of death in the United States."(Journal Epidemiologic Reviews, 2007,29:6-28.cEpub 2007 May 17)

How did we, a nation with a pioneer spirit of activity, determination, perseverance, dedication to hard work, resourcefulness and innovation get to this point of such poor physical fitness and health? Experiencing all of the health robbing diseases of being obese, such as sugar diabetes, high blood pressure, strokes, blood clots and heart disease just to name a few.

Could we as Americans be suffering from the same condition of physical fitness, exercise and health insanity, collectively as a nation, as we are as individuals? As we consider all of the physical fitness gurus who have been making claims for years that they can help us to lose weight, become fit and healthy and keep it off by doing the same old things and using the same old approaches as we have done for many many years and expect a different outcome or result.

For the past 40 years or so we have had an explosion of physical fitness experts that have come on the scene and have claimed that their program is going to make us healthy and lean. As we later participate in their programs we find out that it is just a new version of some already tried boxing, kickboxing, military boot camp, football training camp, or aerobic program that has been tried and failed many times before! If it worked we wouldn't be fat!

Or we are exposed to the next gadget or fad that will help us to shake the weight off, to twist the weight off, to blast the weight off, to burn the weight off, to eat the weight off, or dance the weight off! All the while the weight comes back and is not staying off! As a matter of fact we normally put more weight back on then we had before we started the program! Is that crazy or what?

And we continue to do this over and over and over and over again! We know what happened to us the last time, going up and down just like a yo-yo. Lose weight then we gain the weight again, lose weight then we gain weight again and again and again. We do this weight gain and weight loss dance as if we do not want to change partners or offend our partner or make them mad! The Fat has No Feelings, We Need to Get Rid Of It, Before It Gets Rid Of Us!

It is time for us to stop the madness, the craziness and the insanity and get on the path to a sane, simple, safe, satisfying and successful journey to physical fitness, movement and most of all to great health right now! We have tried so many things and as yet have not found anything that has worked, especially for us or for our nation as a whole. Because if we had we would not be in the poor physical condition that we are presently in as a nation.

But how did we get to this point now and what are we going to do to correct the problem? If you're ready then we want you to join us on this journey to the best and easiest fitness and movement program created just for our nation. Let us welcome you to the future of fitness and movement today, welcome to Sitacise! And let us teach you how to sit & get fit everywhere you might sit.

Before we do that we are going to show you just what happened to us in the past so that we can prevent it from happening to us again in the future. We Americans are too valuable and special to allow ourselves to become obese and suffer from the large assortment of diseases that come with it.

We are better & worth more than that America! And we can win the battle of the bulge individually and as a nation Now!

Chapter 3

Looking Back To The Past To See Our Future!

The Workout:

With our Sitacise Fitness Program we will show you how to get fit anyplace you might sit, but before we do that let's take a look at how we as Americans got into this condition in the first place. Maybe if we take a look at our past and what we used to do and how it affected our health and fitness then, it might help us to correct our present fitness and health problems and provide us with the answers we need now to correct them. All right now let's get ready, let's get set, And Let's Goooo!

One of the most difficult things for us to do is to admit that we have made a mistake and that we are wrong whenever we do make a mistake. For years everyone has held to the belief that if you work out at a prescribed time and at a certain intensity and maintained good healthy eating habits that you would become healthy & fit or be able to maintain your health and fitness if you were already healthy. We always wanted to make sure we planned time to get our daily work out in.

We had to make sure we got to the gym, the park, the studio, the Boys and Girls club or the "Y" to either hit the weights, run the track or do some other kinds of cardio class to make sure we were getting in shape. And we'd better not miss a workout because then we had to do two a days the next day to make up the difference. Man were we dedicated to get the "burn" from lifting those weights or we couldn't wait to get the runner's high from running all those miles. It just seemed like the right thing to do was to work out and to get healthy and fit.

Then we got into the running, jogging craze, we started running 1k then 2k's then 3k's & 5k's and pretty soon we were jogging all over the place. We even had baby strollers that were especially designed to be pushed while we were jogging. And we had those baby carriers that we strapped to our backs or sometimes our fronts as we bounded and bounced down the street getting our jog in. We even wore those that were color-coordinated with the outfit that we had on. Maybe through some strange kind of osmosis the baby would become healthier also.

We started to get good at this jogging thing so we had to take it to the next level didn't we, of course we did. Now everyone and their mother were talking about running a marathon!

It didn't have to be a full marathon like the ones that are over 26 miles, that didn't matter. It just had to have the word *"__Marathon__"* in it!

Because everybody had to know that now we had become serious about this jogging, running thing and now we were going to be

"competing", that we were going to be in a running contest. We were not just your common everyday joggers anymore, we were competitors, we were Marathoners! Yeah man, let's

go out and put in some miles, go and hit the bricks and when we get back go shoot some hoops!

If we weren't into the running thing then we probably got into the power-walking thing, take off those heels, throw on those gym shoes at lunchtime and instead of eating our lunch we were walking baby! We had a nice little course laid out that would allow us to get in those miles we needed so we could burn that fat baby! Takes you back down the old memory lane doesn't it? Almost everyone seemed to be getting in on this fitness craze!

We surely can't forget the aerobic movement can we? We put on our tight spandex color-coordinated outfits, our headbands and our cross trainer shoes (we had to wear cross-trainers because who knew when we might decide to get into something else like a racquetball match or a basketball game). We even scheduled dates at the gym, the saying "meet me at the club after work took on a whole new meaning".

We even begin wearing workout suits as outfits for dates and other events besides working out. Man oh Man we sure did look like we were going to be fit forever! Even rappers were wearing workout clothes and gym shoes when they performed.

We even went through a period of time when people were being robbed & the thief was stealing the victims' athletic shoes!
Some unfortunate individuals were killed over a pair of athletic shoes. It became so bad that individuals started wearing their athletic shoes untied as a signal to the criminals that they were

not going to resist them if they tried to rob them of their athletic shoes. Isn't that hard to believe? Now it seems as if people will try to kill you if you suggest they put on athletic shoes and get a workout! We're just kidding, we're just kidding!

The aerobic movement took the country by storm. It was a physical conditioning program designed to improve one's respiratory and circulatory efficiency. It consisted of doing vigorous activity for sustained periods of time, such as jogging, biking, taking a long swim, power walking, or jumping rope, ect. We had jogging and running clubs, biking clubs, swimming teams, rope jumping teams and power walking clubs, ect.

It seemed as if we would be working out as the old people used to say, " until the cows come home" or for a very long long time. What happened to change all that? What turned things around, well let me tell you but before I do I want to talk to you about another thing that happened on the way to 75% of all Americans being overweight by 2015 in the next chapter!

Chapter 4

What Are You Eating Now?

The Food

The next thing we did was we got into the health food craze and we were counting the calories that were in foods and we were reading food labels on the sides of every thing that we were eating. We're even had labels put on the sides of fast food containers so that we could know what amount of calories we were consuming as we are flying through our favorite fast food joint! We had this great explosion of salad bars opening up and everyone wanted to eat healthy foods.

Then we started to get on all of these crazy and different diets and eating fads. You all know the ones, we went on the eat nothing but only one type of food diet. Kathy and I tried that one and we both went on that diet to lose weight. But instead of losing weight we each gain several pounds! That diet seemed as if it was just too good to be true and it was.

Next we went on a diet that specified that we could only eat a certain type of soup and that diet not only caused us to lose weight but it also kept us going to the bathroom so much that we were afraid that we were going to have to move our beds in there. As a matter of fact we were almost tempted to buy some stock in one of the major toilet paper companies. I want to tell you that that particular diet was one of the biggest pains in the you know where that we have ever experienced.

Next we tried the diet that we only had to be on for several days and then we would get off of it for several days, then we went back on it for several days and this diet was really a very confusing diet and was very easy to forget the days that we were on it and the days that we were off. Plus the main thing as with most diets you really didn't want to be on it anyway. And this diet didn't work either. As with most diets it failed also!

Then we went from eating food to just drinking our food with some of the many variations of the "liquid diets." All of a sudden we didn't have to eat anything, all we had to do was just suck down our food through a straw for breakfast, lunch and dinner. We could throw away our knives, forks, spoons and plates and just carry around a straw and we're ready for dinner. This diet helped to lose a lot of weight but once we started to eat solid foods, we blew up like Santa Claus! That diet didn't work either. It all seems like such a long, long, long time ago doesn't it. We would try anything to lose weights, even if it was unhealthy.

The things that we have been through in terms of dealing with the exercise programs that we have exposed ourselves to and the eating plans that we have subjected ourselves to would be hard to believe if we hadn't live through it ourselves. What a ride! But with all the things that we had attempted to do to stay fit and healthy, How did we become the fatness nation on earth? How Did We Get Here? It's kind of crazy and scary isn't it? WOW!

Chapter 5

How Did We Get Here!

The Process On The Job

With all that has been stated, we still have to answer the question of how did a nation that seemed to be going through what can only be described as a love affair with physical fitness and exercise. A nation that seemed to be so concerned about what it was eating that it would try anything to lose weight, get into the position that it now finds itself in! <u>Being called the fattest nation In the world!</u>

How did this proud America with its great past of hard working, determined, innovative and inventive individuals with as much pride as anyone get to this point of having waistlines that would make Santa Claus envious. Is this a matter of pride? Is this a matter of self-respect, of self-esteem? Or maybe just maybe it is none of those reasons. Maybe it has nothing to do with self-respect, self-esteem or pride. But maybe our ability to be innovative and inventive is the things that got us to this point.

Maybe we were too smart for our own good and for our own good health! How can being innovative and inventive be a bad thing especially when it comes to our health and our waistlines as a nation?

The most important thing that stands out in all of this is that because of our intellectual leadership and our innovative and inventive nature we have been able to create an environment that is unlike any that our forefathers existed in. When our ancestors had to do work they were required to do this most likely from a standing position. From the standing position they normally had to physically do something to perform their jobs.

They had to pick up or lift something up, physically carry it from point A to point Z and then physically put it away. Earlier Americans who were farmers were required to work in a field all day standing and performing physical tasks such as plowing fields, digging in the ground, planting and harvesting crops. They used their bodies and worked long hours standing or bending to perform their various chores. It didn't matter if we were farmers that raised crops, or if we were dairy farmers, or if we were raising cattle for beef, or we did some other kind of physical labor we used our body to perform our jobs.

If we were employed in a factory or plant we had to stand and manufacture something normally for the duration of our eight-hour work shift. Or performs some type of service such as working on an assembly line physically attaching parts and assembling different products while standing. The thing that was required of us while on most jobs was to use our bodies in the performance of our duties while on the job.

Then came automation with its quest to have a machine do what a man used to do. In 1961, General Motors installed the Unimate in a New Jersey factory. Unimate was a robot that was designed to do a welding job on automobile bodies. The Unimate was able to do this task very successfully, so successfully as a matter of fact that this started employers' to look at other jobs that American workers were now doing that machines could do.

This caused many other factories to begin installing robots in their own facilities.

Industrial robots began performing a variety of human duties such as assembling, sealing, welding, sorting, material handling and many other jobs previously performed by humans. It wasn't long before robots and machines were also being designed to do some of the other jobs that American workers had been doing such as painting, counting, inspecting and many other jobs that were previously performed by American workers.

The robots were doing a lot of the physical jobs and were replacing human beings and now we humans, (Americans), were either monitoring the robots as they performed their jobs or had been replaced by the robots and lost our physical jobs altogether. American workers who had up to this time been working these physical jobs, were now going for more additional training and getting more education to become qualified to get less physical technical jobs or office or desk jobs.

Americans started to seek this kind of job or career path and going to school with a thought in mind of receiving the type of education that would allow them to become qualified to do less physical jobs. Colleges, Universities & technical schools begin to see their attendance increase as Americans hurried to receive training for jobs that offer the opportunity to do less physical labor. We were encouraging everyone to pursue an education so that *"they would not get stuck in a plant, factory or some other place that required us to do physical labor!"* It was as if as a nation we were saying that physical labor, physical jobs and even doing physical things were not as important as pursuing our education and getting a less physical job and leading a less physical life. We seemed to slowly becoming a nation in transition, instead of relying upon ourselves we were more dependent upon automation to do it for us and we were content in letting that happen.

There were also other great benefits to becoming more increasingly dependent upon robots and machines to do the job for us. Robots and machines do not need sick pay, vacations hospitalization or days off. They don't need to rest or take lunch breaks and they're not always complaining about the working conditions or the boss or management. The robots or the machines will work as much over time as the bosses require them to without one complaint, just give it some oil & minor repairs.

I only mention this because this is why there is a great incentive for all employers to incorporate as many robots and machines within the manufacturing process as is possible. But when this was done it took away from the American workers more physical job opportunities thus preventing the American workers from using their bodies to move in a physical way, for eight hours per day, five days per week or more.

In summary what occurred during this period of automation in factories and plants, combined with the fact that the American psyche was now geared toward performing less physical jobs; was the loss of at least 40 hours per week of physically moving, using our bodies while on the job for many American worker! That's A Lot of Hours of Physical Movement Lost per Week!

Many companies began to outsource American jobs to other countries. Outsourcing is a process sending American jobs to foreign countries and foreign labor to perform physical or undesirable jobs that Americans had done and now were no longer doing. This practice eliminated many of the physical jobs that we Americans traditionally did and now are not doing.

This is another loss of physical activity & movement that we Americans were doing that we are no longer doing. Slowly we are doing less and less physical activity, less physical movement, less calories burned from doing less of those movements.

THINK ABOUT IT AMERICA!

Chapter 6

The Process

Automation in The Home

Along with automation on the job there was increased automation now in the American home. It was no longer necessary for us Americans to wash our families clothing by hand or even have to go outside to hang the clothes on the line to dry. Now we have a washer and dryer that could do that for us. The hours that we used to use to physically wash those clothes by hand and stand up and hang them on the line and remove them from the line when they dried was no longer necessary. Now it only takes us a few minutes to load and unload the washer and dryer. Then we go sit somewhere and watch something.

We used to take those dry cloths off the line one at a time and fold them and place them in a basket while we were standing up on washday. Often times we would be talking to our neighbor about the neighborhood gossip as we were *standing there* folding our cloths together. Then we would physically pick up our baskets of cloths and carry them into the house and *walk* to wherever they needed to be taken to and physically put them down or away. No wonder they called it washed day back then because it took almost all day to do it.

We have ranges with ovens that have a brain and can even thaw foods out, cook the food and tell us when it is done. All we have to do is spend a little time to prepare the food for cooking and it will do the rest. We have other conveniences that our family can use without having to use their bodies as much and as long to perform these tasks. Talk about the good life!

We Americans no longer have to stand at the sink for about 30 minutes to an hour to wash and dry dishes now we have a dishwasher that can wash the dishes for us. Instead of standing up to wash and dry dishes we can now just take a few minutes to load the dishwasher and wait for the dishes to be washed and dried for us. We don't even have to scrape the dishes anymore because of the pot scrubber features. Man do we have it made!

We now have the microwave that can make our meals at lightning speed. This also caused the creation of many different microwavable meals. Now we needed faster meal preparation options because we were busy pursuing more training and education needed to get one of those less physical demanding jobs and now we don't have time to prepare our meals in the traditional manner. It just was too time-consuming. Let's just pop it in the microwave and nuke that sucker! It was fast, it was convenient and it got us to our next class, appointment or job on time. Got to make haste, no time to waste!

It did not matter that we may never have heard of some of the ingredients in those microwavable creations and concoctions that we were throwing into that microwave. What was important is that it was quick and fast and helped to keep our lives moving at this super-fast pace that we were now on trying to get our education, work on a job and have a little time for recreation.

The fast food phenomena is now upon us because we decided that it not only was convenient to microwave our foods but now we could get a complete dinner prepared for us by someone else and we could get it done fast! It was so interesting because now the family could choose many different offerings for dinner time that mother or the family did not have to cook. They could now order a full six and seven course meal or something as simple as a hamburger and order of french fries without having to lift a finger!

The family didn't have to do the physical movements required to go to the grocery store select the kinds of foods that they we're going to use to prepare the meal. They didn't have to walk to the car, drive to the store, get out of the car, walked to the store, walked down the aisles, select and pick up the food, place it in the cart, walk to the checkout and pay for the food, walk back to the car, unload the groceries into the car, drive the car back home, unload the groceries from the car, walk to the house with the groceries, put away the groceries, prepare the meal, serve the meal, and then finally clean up after the meal.

Someone else was now doing all of the physical activities that we used to perform when we were performing the simple tasks associated with of preparing a meal for the family, for us. Did you realize that it requires so many steps and that we had performed so much movement when we were preparing a meal?

Because we were now so busy pursuing a career with a desk job and maybe a corner office in the picture somewhere, if we had any children we now could hire a babysitter or take them to a day care. No longer were we performing the tasks of raising our children, such as playing with them daily or preparing their meals or taking them on little walks or trips to the playground or even the little things such as watching them and keeping them out of trouble or getting into mischief. As anyone knows that has had to take care of or baby-sit any children no matter what the age, it is a task that requires a lot of physical and mental activity.

There are also many school programs that offer babysitting services or day care services in the form of head start or other type programs of this kind that will allow the parents to drop off the child and someone else will expend their physical energy caring for and providing meals for the parent's child.

This is not automation but part of the process of becoming educated to participate in the automation process. This is also another example of how Americans have another decrease in the amount of physical movement that we now participate in during our lives. This is not condemnation for these day cares or child caring services, or the people that use them, it just points out one more task that we no longer physically participate in that we used to participate in.

We don't even wrestle or rough house with our children as we used to when we were children. If we have a child that is very active as we were as children we are now calling them hyper active and we will medicate them to slow them down! We need to let them *"as the old folk use to say let them run off some steam and let them get tuckered out."* We bet it's been along time since you heard that phrase. But let's not slow down, we must move on to the next chapter. We Know You're Busy! Got to keep moving to the next place to sit!

Chapter 7

The Process Automation in the Home

The Television

If we recall our history correctly, the television was invented by John Logie Baird, a Scottish engineer and inventor, in Hastings, England in 1923. As these living moving images were later carried electronically by the BBC as it began the first television broadcasts in the world in 1929. Never in his wildest dreams could Mr. Baird have anticipated the popularity of his invention. With almost religious fervor people gather to worship at his shrine every day. And unlike most worshipers, his devotees seem to never miss a service!

In the 1950s color television was introduced and that made those moving images appear even more lifelike to its viewers. As time marched on and the improvements to the televisions were so lifelike that the viewer now feels as if he is experiencing the program for himself. With the improvements to the sound systems and picture quality, it is almost as if the program is being lived out right in the viewer's home!

Along with the improvements of the television sets especially with the addition of the remote control, Americans began to watch more and more television. Because of the remote control we Americans do not even have to expend the physical energy needed to get up and turn the channel. We can sit down and even do that. Now we can watch the television in total couch potato bliss, almost like being in couch potato heaven.

In the Nielsen Media Research's latest report, the average American household watches eight hours and 15 minutes of television in a 24-hour period. The report went on to state that the average amount of time for individuals that are over two years of age, is about 4 1/2 hours per day. Now that is a lot of TV viewing! A lot of sitting & doing little physical movement time!

This should be looked at with the understanding that there are some individual homes whose viewers may just turn on the television as soon as they come home and they may be busy doing other things besides viewing the television and not watching a program all the time that the television is on.

They may be utilizing the television as convenient background noise as they go about doing other tasks in the other parts of the home and may only occasionally peek in on the television to view it when something of interest comes on.

There are other viewers that may turn on the television set and view a program while they may be performing activities such as running on the treadmill at home or working out on their elliptical trainer or on a stationary bicycle or some other type of physical fitness equipment. There are weightlifters that like to turn on the television and work out while they are watching a lifting routine that is being televised.

We have also spoken with people who like to turn on their favorite cooking program and prepare their family's meal for that evening while watching one of the many celebrities cooking programs that are now so popular on television. So there are exceptions that need to be considered when we look upon the total time that's being used to watch television and not perform any physical activity or movement.

One of the major concerns that has been voiced about too much television watching is that the viewer may become addicted just as with any other addiction. In an article by Stefan Anitei, dated December 14, 2007 on m.softpedia.com, the question was asked would you give up watching TV forever for $1 million and 25% of the Americans who were asked the question said no. In another study men were asked what would make them happy and the main wish was a plasma TV!

In the March 2007 Center for Disease Control Study titled, Reducing Children's TV Time to Reduce the Risks of Childhood Overweight: The Children's Media Use Study. It was reported that on average the children had screen time of nearly 5 1/2 hours per day. The recommendation from the study was for the children to have no more than 2 hours of screen time from all sources that included TVs, computers and video games. When choosing their favorite activities the children listed some type of media as being their favorite activity almost 75% of the time. They listed a physical activity about 25% of the time. The fear is that there will be even more physical activity hours wasted on watching TV, computers and video games.

Chapter 8

The Process Automation in The Home

The Personal Home Computer

In the early 1970s there was something that was created that really changed the landscape and made a difference in the lives of so many Americans forever. This was the big one, the EL GRANDE MUCHO! It changed the way that many of the physical activities that Americans had previously performed would now be done forever! When this device was first introduced into the home it was touted as a solution to many of the tasks that we performed in the home. It did not disappoint.

This item was to provide us with the ability to do everything from managing the family budget to providing endless hours of recreation for everyone in the family. As this device evolved it became a source for endless information and entertainment but also a tremendous time consumer that Americans now spend countless hours with. This device is our "Personal Home Computers"! Man do we get up close & personal with it!

This is a device that has eliminated so much physical movement that we used to do that we will only make mention of a few of them here. As we consider the computer and its great ability to do many things to simplify our lives we must note within the simplification process there are many physical movements that the personal computer now does for us and that we no longer have to do for ourselves.

When we began to consider something as simple as e-mailing our fellow workers on the job. In the past if we wanted to speak with one of our fellow employees we might call them up and then walked down to their office or cubicle to speak with them. Now we contact him by e-mail even if they're only a few steps away and converse with them. Or we chat with them on the computer.

This also includes text messaging from our personal telephone computers. We may even be in the same crowded room but we are busy texting each other. In the past we may have decided to take a walk and converse with each other to get away from the crowd in the room. But with text messaging we can have a private conversation in the midst a crowded room full of many people.

In the past when we wanted to pay a bill we would get the bill, write a check for it and take it down to the post office and mail the bill. Or we would get the bill and go to the establishment where we had to pay the bill and pay the bill by check or charge. Now we have the convenience of paying that bill online. We do not have to perform the physical activity of going to the post office or the establishment and stand in line and wait to pay our bill.

If we decide that we would like to go shopping we can now go browsing online for everything from a pair of exercise shoes to our next wife or husband. We do not have to get up, get dressed jump in our automobile and go through the process of shopping if we do not choose to. We can do it all online! If we want a new or used car, we can check out the inventory online. Need some medication just go online and get our prescription filled. Whatever we want to buy is no more than a click away.

If we want to get more training or if we want to go to a college or university to get a degree now almost every college or university offers online courses that we can take in our pajamas from the comfort of our own bedrooms in our own homes. We don't even have to bother to get up and clean up to go to our classes! And if we are searching for any kind of information for an assignment. We no longer have to walk down to the library and search through the aisles for books because with the Internet the information is at our fingertips.

In 1972 Magnavox released Odyssey as a home video game, it was the first home video game console ever created. The genie was out of the bottle in regards to home video games now becoming one of the most popular forms of recreation and entertainment that the world has ever seen! They were going to be played on the home computer. It would become the main source of recreation and entertainment in the home.

There are now very complicated and lifelike video games that are so realistic that the participants' report they feel as if they are actually participating in real life events. Because of this phenomenon, this feeling of actually being a participant in the games, many individual that play video games have a great tendency of overindulging in the games and becoming addicted to them. There are reports of people who have neglected to pay their bills and get their much-needed sleep because they were playing video games. Some will even come home from working 12 hour shifts and jump online and play some new multiplayer games for another six or seven hours straight!

And this practice of playing video games for hours is being passed along to our younger generation so much that now its to the point of this being the primary source of their entertainment and recreational activity. Often times along with increased video game playing comes the increased opportunity for more snacking and impulsive eating! In the past this time was used for other physical activities such as playing ball games or walking and visiting with friends or going to the playground for some type of physical movement.

In that same 2007 study about reducing children's screen time, the children were asked to draw a picture of their favorite activity and one participant drew a picture of herself watching a program on the screen while her mother brought her a snack!

In the past mothers use to encourage their children to get out of the house and go play outside and *"work up an appetite."* When the last time we worked up an appetite? And when it was time to eat the mother would call the child in from playing and then the child would eat something because it was hungry! This is just another example of how automation has decreased Americans physical movement and also provides an opportunity for increased caloric input as well.

The television, the personal computer and video games have turned large amounts of our recreation and leisure time into *"lazy time" and pig out time!"* We need to remember that food is The Fuel That Our Bodies Use To Function On, Not Just A Source of Enjoyment. It Provides Us With Energy To Live.

WE MUST EAT TO LIVE, NOT LIVE TO EAT! Fat is store food (glucose) that our bodies didn't need to use for fuel right now; so our bodies stored it as fat to use it later when needed. Our problem is that we tend to eat before we burn up the stored energy that we already have on our bodies. This causes us to become overweight. Lets try to burn up our stored energy before we eat more energy.

Chapter 9

The Process: Inactivity Physiology What's Wrong With Me Sitting So Long?

"I'm grown, I can do what I want If I want to sit and play video games all day, that's my choice"! I'll sit as long as I want Too!

We are sure that we have all heard someone defiantly say that whenever they have been told that a certain activity is not good for them. We recall many times when we heard smokers that said the same thing 20 or 30 years ago and defiantly blew a puff of smoke in our faces or in our direction. We knew that it was not healthy for them or us but they were still able to smoke in public places, have their own section in the restaurants to smoke in and even have designated places inside of their working establishment that they were permitted to smoke in.

Now all of that has changed because we all understand that there are serious health risks involved in being in the same area as someone who is smoking and breathing in all of those chemicals that are associated with secondhand smoke. Some environments are now totally smoke free and we are not even permitted to smoke on the property. That means in the buildings, on the grounds or even in the parking lot!

For many years people tried to drink and drive and they felt as if it was their right and their privilege to do so. They also believed that they were the best to judge how drunk or incapacitated they were. Now we know that there have been many accidents and loss of life caused by drunken drivers and there are laws designed to protect us from these individuals.

We now have much more knowledge and information about the dangers associated with smoking and drinking. Therefore we have taken steps to protect ourselves from the dangers associated with these behaviors and the individuals that indulge in them. We believe that the consumer has a right to know about risks associated with the products that they use. We should be able to make an informed decision about the things that we use or things we do.

There is now a lot more information available about our health, the foods we eat, movement & fitness then ever before.
We have learned that sitting for long periods of time poses many major health risks and that it

effects the body in many negative ways. There is a new field of study called Inactivity Physiology; this field of study is showing a remarkable connection between sitting for long periods and higher rates of diabetes, obesity, heart disease, blood clots, DVT, PE and even mortality.

A study earlier this year in the American Journal of Epidemiology followed 123,000 adults for over 14 years; those who sat for more than 6 hours a day were at least 18% more likely to die sooner than those who sit less than 3 hours a day.

"Sitting is hazardous. It's dangerous. We are on the cusp of a major revolution about what we think of as healthy behavior in the workplace," Marc Hamilton, a leading researcher on inactivity physiology at the Pennington

Biomedical Research Center in Louisiana. He calls sitting the new smoking.

In a recent paper titled, Too Little Exercise and To Much Sitting: Inactivity Physiology And The Need For New Recommendations On Sedentary Behavior, Current cardiovascular risk reports, vol. 2, no. 4, pp. 292-298. A research team of Marc T. Hamilton, Genevieve N. Healy, David W. Dunstan, Theodore W. Zderic and Neville Owens summarized their research findings as follows: "moderate to vigorous intensity physical activity has an established preventive role in cardiovascular disease, type 2 diabetes, obesity, and some cancers. However, recent epidemiologic evidence suggests that sitting time has deleterious cardiovascular and metabolic effects that are independent of whether adults meet physical activity guidelines.

Evidence from "inactivity physiology" laboratory studies has identified unique mechanisms that are distinct from the biologic bases of exercise. Opportunities for sedentary behaviors are ubiquitous and are likely to increase with further innovations of technologies. We present a compelling selection of emerging evidence on the deleterious effects of sedentary behavior, as it is underpinned by the unique physiology of inactivity.

It is time to consider excessive sitting a serious health hazard, with the potential for ultimately giving consideration to the inclusion of too much sitting (or too few breaks from sitting) in physical activity and health guidelines".

To break their findings down into terms that we can easily understand, the researchers have concluded that sitting for too long of a period of time, without any breaks from sitting, would become subtly harmful to our health. As we develop more technical jobs that are and will be everywhere, being inactive will negatively affect our cardiovascular health; increase our risk of sugar diabetes and increase obesity.

The American heart Association's rapid access journal report entitled Sedentary TV Time May Cut Life Short had these findings: the study found that every hour spent in front of the television per day brings with it an 11% greater risk of premature death from all causes, and an 18% greater risk of dying from cardiovascular disease. The findings apply to both obese and overweight people as well as people with a healthy weight because prolonged periods of sitting have an unhealthy influence on blood sugar and blood fat levels. Compared with people who watch less than 2 hours of television daily, those who watch more than 4 hours a day had a 46% higher risk of death from all causes & an 80% increase risks for CVD-related deaths.

This association held regardless of other independent and common cardiovascular disease risk factor, including smoking, high blood pressure, high blood cholesterol, unhealthy diet, excessive waist circumference, and leisure time exercises. "The human body was designed to move, not to sit for extended periods of time", said David Dunstan, Ph.D., the study's lead author and professor and head of the Physical Activities Lavatory in the Division of Metabolism and Obesity at the Baker IDI

Heart and Diabetes Institute in Victoria, Australia.

"What has happened is that a lot of the normal activities of daily living that involves standing up &moving the muscles in the body had been converted to sitting," Dunstan said. "Technological, social, and economic changes mean that people don't move their muscles as much as they used to-consequently the levels of energy expenditure people use to go about their lives continues to shrink. For many people on a daily basis they shift from one chair to another-from the chair in the car-to the chair at work-to the chair in front of the television." Dunstan said.

In a 2010 study in the Journal of Applied Physiology it was found that when healthy men limited the number of footsteps by 85% for two weeks, they experienced a 17% decrease in insulin sensitivity, raising their diabetes risk. That is For Only 2 Weeks!

Recently I spoke with a young man that I had not seen for several years. He had gained over 40 pounds and he began to explain to me why he had gained so much weight. He said that he had inherited an automobile and that the places that he had previously walked to he now was driving to them, even the close places. He said that the weight came on slowly and over a period of about three years and that he had gained it at a rate of about 11/2 pounds per month.

He also explained because he was now able to get to places a lot faster than he had before he had the car, he now had more time on his hands and he was sitting around a whole lot more than he ever had before. He has decided to lose the weight because of his looks and his health. He is now going to incorporate more walking and Sitacise exercises into his daily routine and stop being so dependent on his automobile.

As we can see from all of the different examples that we have cited, sitting for long periods of time, puts we Americans at risk of experience more heart attacks, having more sugar diabetes, increased risks of getting some forms of cancer and especially increases our chances of being obese. It does that to us regardless of our being normal weight, overweight or obese. And regardless of how much exercise we may be getting! We must incorporate more movement into our normal daily activities. We cannot just limits our working out or exercising to just a specific period of time but we must incorporate more movement into our regular daily activities!

Don't just sit in that seat, get fit in that seat!

Chapter 10

Sitting Disease: The New Epidemic

According to a poll of 6300 people that was conducted by the Institute for Medicine and Public Health, it was discovered that the average American spends almost 56 hours a week sitting working at a computer screen, driving our cars, or flipping through the channels looking at our high definition television.

The study revealed that women are more sedentary then men, since they play fewer sports than men and also hold less active jobs. "Our bodies have evolved over millions of years to do one thing: move," says James Levine. M.D. Ph.D. of the Mayo Clinic in Rochester, Minnesota. "As human beings, we evolved to stand upright. For thousand generations, our environment demanded nearly constant physical activity.

"When we sit for extended periods of time, our bodies start to shut down at the metabolic level, when muscles, especially those big ones meant for movement, the gluteus maximus, hamstrings and quadriceps are immobile, our circulation slows and we burn fewer calories. Key flab or fat burning enzymes that are responsible for breaking down triglycerides simply start switching off. Sit for full day and those fat burners plummet by 50%", Levine says.

That's not all. The less we move, the less blood sugar our bodies use; research showed that for every two hours spent on our back side per day, our chances of contracting diabetes goes up 7%. We're also more prone to depression because with less blood flow-fewer feel-good hormones are circulating to our brains. Does the words *"brain fog"* ring a bell? People that do Sitacise regularly reported that they feel a lot more alert and mentally sharp on those days that they did it. One of the most often heard responses is that after Sitacise, I Feel Alive!

Persons that we questioned about Sitacise reported that on the days of doing Sitacise they are more energetic on the job and perform the functions of the job a lot easier then on the days that they don't do Sitacise. They explained that they felt as if they can handle any challenge that the job, their boss and their fellow workers could dish out to them that day! One excited worker said, on those days, "I feel like I can take on the world and win."

Have you ever watched a group of children enjoying the simple exercise of running? We work with children of varied social economical backgrounds and age groups instructing them in physical fitness and exercise. We have observed the children running relays and have witnessed them having so much fun and being excited about competing with and beating their peers in these relay races. They have great spirit and enthusiasm while they are participating in these races and it easy to see that we human beings and Americans were made to move and not to sit.

We also have the children participate in other moving activities such as calisthenics, games of dodge ball, kickball, competitive dribbling, ect. and the children just love to move. In some of our classes we have teachers participate that are slightly more mature than me and I'm 58!

There just seems to be something inside of all of us humans and Americans that comes alive when we are given the opportunity to move. We believe, as the researchers do that there is something extremely unnatural about us Americans sitting for long periods of time as we do now!

In a Men's Health issue, updated 10/26/'10, by Maria Masters, the question was asked; do you lead and active or sedentary lifestyle? Paraphrasing the article, it stated that if you were a busy person that worked 60 hours per week but still managed to get 5-45 minute workouts in you would be considered to be active by most experts' standards. But according to researcher Marc Hamilton, Ph.D. you would be considered to be an exercising couch potato. Hamilton stated, "people tend to view physical activity on a single continuum." "On the far side you have people who exercise a lot and on the other you have people who don't exercise at all, but they're not polar opposites"

"A new growing body of research is showing that the amount of time you spend on your butt sitting and the amount of time you spend exercising are completely separate factors for heart disease risk. And the new research also suggests that the more hours per day that we sit, the greater our likelihood of dying an earlier death regardless of how much we exercise or how lean we are. That's right: even a sculpted six-pack can't protect you from your chair"; the article continued.

"But it's not just your heart that is at risk from too much sitting; your hips, spine and shoulders could also suffer. In fact, sitting can ruin you from head to toe." The article explained.

Remember the study in the Journal of Applied Physiology that found when healthy men limited their number of footsteps by 85% for just two weeks, they experienced a 17% decrease in insulin sensitivity, raising the diabetes risk."

Peter Katzmarzyk, Ph.D, Hamilton's colleague at Pennington, the nation's leading obesity research Center, said, "that regularly exercising is not the same as being active." Official exercise activity, such as running, or weightlifting, are different then so-called non-exercise activities, like walking to our car or cutting our grass. A person may hit the gym every day, <u>but if he is sitting a good deal of the</u>

rest of the time, he probably is not leading an overall active life," says Katzmarzyk.

In a 2007 reports, University of Missouri scientists said that people with the highest levels of non-exercise activity (those who did little to no actual exercise) burned significantly more calories a week then those who ran 35 miles a week but accumulated only a moderate amount of nonexercise activity. This could result in as much as a person that does less nonexercise activity burning 500 to a thousand less calories a day. This could translate into gaining as much as 16 pounds in eight months to a year," the article reported.

We don't know about you but that seems like a lot of weight to us in a short period of time, but the article goes on to reveal even more very significant factors. In 2009 Katzmarzyk studied the lifestyle habits of more than 17,000 men and women and found that those who sat for almost the entire day were 54% more likely to have a heart attack than those who sat almost none of the time! It didn't matter how much sitters weighed, how often they exercised or if they did or didn't smoke. Sitting is an independent risk factor.

In 1953 British study, scientists examined 2 groups of workers: bus drivers and trolley conductors. The bus driver sat their entire day; the trolley conductors were running up and down the stairs and aisles of the double decker trolleys. Neither group did any other exercise. As it turned out the bus drivers were nearly twice as likely to die of heart disease as the conductors were. TWICE AS LIKELY!

Hamilton studied how exercise affects an enzyme called lipoprotein lipase (LPL). LPL's main responsibility is to break down fat in the bloodstream to use it as energy. If the enzyme doesn't work in our legs the fat is stored instead of burned as fuel. When sitting for long uninterrupted periods of time the activity of the LPL decreases significantly but when there is more activity the activity of the LPL increases tenfold. "We must treat the problem specifically," Hamilton stated. We must stop sitting for such long uninterrupted periods of time and we need to get up and move.

That is why we created Sitacise to get sedentary persons moving every six minutes so that the LPL can do its job of burning blood sugars and blood fats and not storing them as fats. But there is more to this *"sitting disease"* that we will cover in the next chapter because sitting for long periods of time has many hidden dangers that we as the American public need to

know about so we can make informed decisions about our health, exercise, fitness & jobs.

Chapter 11

Sitting Disease

Sit in the Chair Become the Chair

"Your body adapts to what you do most often, says Bill Hartman, P. T., C.S.C.S., a physical therapists in Indianapolis, Indiana. "So if you sit in a chair all day, you've essentially become better adapted to sitting in a chair. "The trouble is that makes you less adept at standing, walking, running, and jumping, all of which a truly healthy human being should be able to do with proficiency. "Older folks have a hard time moving around then younger people do," says Hartman. "That's not simply because of age; it's because what we do consistently from day to day manifest itself over time, for good and bad."

When we examine Mr. Hartman's words he is simply stating that if we indulge in good healthy physical activities and we make it a habit to do those things, that we are going to find that we are more capable of doing those physical activities. If we make it a habit of sitting for long periods of time and not perform any physical activities it won't be long before we will become good at not being able to do any physical activities. And not only will we become good at not performing any of those physical activities, we'll also began to believe that we cannot perform those activities. Sit in the Chair, Become the Chair!

Why did we mention believing, because it is important that we have the right attitude when we start any change in our lives. We must start believing that we can do more physical activity while at work, such as Sitacise, so that we can undo the negative affects of long uninterrupted periods of sitting. A positive attitude will help us get very positive results! Let's start thinking like the winners that we are and we will win this battle of the bulge!

When we sat all day at our desks in recent jobs at a call center that we had, we noticed some very troubling things that happened to Kathy's body. Mark did Sitacise on the job and moved at least every 6 minutes for at least 30 seconds and had very little pain or stiffness and no weight gain. Kathy was not as lucky. Her muscles became very stiff after sitting for about 35-45 continuous minutes. She experienced pain in her lower back, neck, hips, gluteus maximus, and had pain in her tailbone area. She exercised on the job sporadically, about 6 minutes per 8 hour shift. She also gained 8 pounds in 9 weeks.

The reason why this occurs is that the fascia, a tough connective tissue that covers all our muscles tends to set in the position that our muscles are most often in. So if we sit most of the time, our fascia adopts to that specific position! "When we sit our hips and thighs are bent, this causes the muscles on the front of thighs, our hip flexors to shorten. The more we sit the more our fascia will keep our hip flexors shortened," says Hartman. "This condition causes us to walk with a foreword lean, the muscles don't stretch as they naturally should. Instead of walking tall and straight our fascia has adapted more to sitting than standing" he went on to say.

Simply put the more time that we spend in a chair, the more our bodies adapt to that position and the more we look as if we have spent time sitting in the chair. While we were working at this call center it was quite noticeable that many people were suffering from this condition.

"If we spend a lot of time with our shoulders and upper back slump over a keyboard, this becomes our normal posture. This can lead to chronic neck and shoulder pain. If we like to sit with our legs crossed we may experience hip imbalances, which makes our lower body less stable. This decreases agility and athletic performance and increases our risk for injuries." A person who sits a lot becomes less efficient in everything they do that involves moving", says Hartman.

"Our gluteus maximus, medius and minimus
or our butt muscles are our body's largest
muscle group. If we sit on them too much they
will forget how to fire or work." This is a
condition called "gluteal amnesia," and if they
don't work properly our bodies loses our biggest
muscle for burning blood sugars and blood
fats," he continued. We also will be less able to
lift our bodies or our weight when we squat or
bend down to pick up something.

Mark was doing Sitacise legwork that
engaged the gluteus muscles at least every 12
minutes while working. This permitted him not
only to keep these muscles strong, but also
assisted in his not gaining any additional weight
while working in the call center. Because when
he did our Sitacise movements his large gluteus
muscles, quadricep muscles, adductor, abductor,

calf muscles, shins, hamstrings and abdominal muscles were being contracted and engaged so often.

"When we have weak gluteus maximus muscles as well as tight hip flexors our pelvis will tilt forward. This puts stress on our lumbar spine resulting in low back pain. It also pushes our bellies out and gives us a protruding stomach look even if we don't have an ounce of fat." "These changes are subtle at first but over time they will begin to get worse and are a lot harder to fix," continued Hartman.

Mark and Kathy noticed many individuals whose body types would fit this description that worked at the call center. There were workers that were overweight and had potbellies. There were also others that had potbellies without being overweight. Other workers also have that foreword body lean and walk as if they were going to tip over and fall on their faces. Most of the workers that we spoke with about exercise and fitness seem to be completely unaware that these conditions could be the results of having weak gluteus maximus muscles and tighter hip flexors. Of those whom we spoke to they just thought that it was necessary for them to lose weight and get in shape through traditional exercises.

Kathy had introduced several of the workers to our Sitacise exercises and they were doing them sporadically while they were working. Kathy had just spoken with them about the aspects of weight gain when sitting for long periods of time but she did not have the opportunity for us to come in and cover the other dangers associated with sitting for long uninterrupted periods of time.

The report illustrated that we know there is a gene in the body that causes heart disease, but it doesn't respond to exercise no matter how often or hard we work out, and yet the activity of the gene becomes worse from sitting because of the complete and utter lack of contractile activity in our muscles. The more non-exercise movements we do, the more nontraditional movements we do while sitting that's the real cure. We need to look at the time that we sit in our chairs and work as the time to get in those non-traditional exercise movements so that we are not forfeiting our health for a paycheck.

Mark always says, if we don't have our health we will spend everything that we have to get it; but if we do have our health we can enjoy everything that we have because we've got it! We believe that if all American knew just about these health risk alone, that are associated with sitting for long uninterrupted periods, that we have shown so far; that they would opt to do our Sitacise exercises to eliminate these risks. But sadly there are still more health problems associated with sitting that we will reveal in the rest of the book. Hold on it gets worse!

Chapter 12

Sitting Disease

What a Pain in The B_ _ _!

I bet you noticed that something is missing in the title of this chapter and if you were to say that it is the three letters behind the B you would be right! But if you can tell us what those last three letters are, we will give you $50 billion! Psych! We are only kidding, we're just playing with you but if we had it we would give it to you! Sure We Would! Sure We Would!

But the reason why those three letters on this chapter are missing is because they represent two different sets of three letters. The first set of letters is ack or the word is Back and we will discuss the back pains that are associated with long periods of uninterrupted sitting and their causes. This will not be an exhaustive discussion but it will be a thorough one that will illustrate many of the back problems and back pains that are commonly encountered during long periods of uninterrupted sitting. It will surprise you what a _**pain in the back**_ sitting can be.

" Disc ruptures occur when the inner portion of the disc protrudes, putting pressure on the nerve roots leading from the spine. Numbness or pain in the legs is a common symptom of ruptured discs in the lower back. This condition is also aggravated by sitting." Disc erosion occurs from continued pressure on the spinal discs, which caused them to become permanently compressed," Mark reported.

"Forceful movements that do not cause harm with one motion, but which can build up a micro-trauma over time. For example, the force generated by sitting for extended periods of time without moving to take a break or alternate positions is a risk factor for low back pain," he continued. "Too much repetition or too little can contribute to micro-trauma, repeated twisting to reach the phone or sitting with the back bent forward can over time lead to ruptured discs."

"Patellofemoral syndrome is another common cause of legs pain while sitting. We will feel pain under and around our kneecap. The pain can get worse when we're active or sitting and we can have it in one knee or both knees," he said.

Because this condition is located in our legs and the pain is under the kneecap, often times we think that it is a leg injury and not due to our sitting. We tend to think we injured it doing something else unrelated to our prolonged uninterrupted sitting. It is very important for us to know that it could be and maybe is related to our sitting. This is why we are writing this book because we want all Americans to understand about the dangers associated with prolonged uninterrupted periods of sitting!

Now we will look briefly at the other letters that this chapter started without and they are the old gluteus maximus, the utt was missing or the butt. One of the other problems with sitting for long periods of time is that it causes sciatic nerve impingement also called sciatica. Sciatica occurs when swelling or tension in certain muscles in the buttocks can put pressure on the sciatic nerve causing pain down the leg.

Mark was involved in a car wreck a few years ago and he suffered from sciatica, it was so painful that it caused him to walk bent over and crooked. He learned a lot about the back and how to treat back pain and then how to prevent the pain from happening again from some of the best back specialists in the world.

He learned that the spine is a series of bones that have small discs that are filled with jellylike substance that acts as shock absorbers between the bones. When the discs are damaged they may bulge or rupture and this jellylike substance can leak out. When this happens we have a disc that we say has been ruptured or slipped. This condition can cause tingling or numbness in one leg that begins at the buttock and extends to the ankle or foot. It can also cause weakness in the muscles of one or both legs. It can also lead to the loss of bladder and/or bowel control from nerve root compression called cauda equina syndrome. We can also have deep muscle pain and muscle spasms when we have a ruptured disc.

When we sit for long periods of time on our buttocks they usually rest on the ischial tuberosity. This is the most common cause of pain at the cheek line in the buttock area. This can also be called ischial bursitis that is so painful that any pressure on the involved bursa would have the affected individual literally "hit the ceiling in pain!" This pain is normally worse the first thing in the morning.

There is another injury that can result from sitting for long periods of time it is called coccydynia. It is the inflammation of one area, the bottom of the tailbone or coccyx. It causes pain and tenderness in that area and is worsened by sitting. Kathy has this injury because of her prolonged sitting at the call center. She has learned to make adjustments in her sitting positions by changing them frequently and not sitting in the same position for long uninterrupted periods of time.

As we can see there are many different back and butt problems we can experience by sitting for long uninterrupted periods of time. This is not an exhaustive look at all of the back and butt problems that we can experience while sitting for long uninterrupted periods of time, but it definitely does let us realize the great danger that our bodies are exposed to when we sit for long uninterrupted periods of time. We will explore the solutions to this problem later on in the book, but right now we're going to examine some the problems that our legs experience when we sit for long uninterrupted periods of time.

Chapter 13

The Sitting Disease (Epidemic!)
My Legs Are Killing Me!

If we start to have or have had pains in our legs such as tenderness and swelling of the calf or if our calves become warm and red, we may be suffering from a condition called Deep Vein Thrombosis or (DVT). It is also called "the economy class syndrome." People who sit through long airplane flights without moving around can develop blood clots in veins deep within their lower leg or thighs, reports the National Institute of Health in its July 2007 News in Health publication titled, Recognize and Prevent Deep Vein Thrombosis.

The paper informed it's not just airplane flights that raise our risk but anyone sitting in a car, at a desk or elsewhere for long periods of time without moving is at high risk. DVT can cause serious complications if not treated however, only half of the people with DVT have symptoms. That is why it is so important for us to be taking precautionary measures of doing movements such as those in our Sitacise program so that we can be proactive and ensure that we are moving and not sitting for long uninterrupted periods of time.

The above-mentioned symptoms usually appear in only one leg and we might only feel the leg pain when we are standing or walking. It is important to see a doctor right away if you have these symptoms, the paper continued. Some people find out that they have DVT only after the clot is moved from the leg and traveled to the lungs and develops into a pulmonary embolism.

If the clot is small we may not even notice it as it flows through our blood system undetected because of its size and because it is too tiny to become lodged in our veins. If we experience shortness of breath and chest pains when we take a deep breath, that could be a sign of a medium pulmonary embolism that has traveled to our lungs and is lodged there. A large pulmonary embolism can cause collapse and even sudden death!

It is also reported that those who have had one episode of DVT are at greater risk of having another blood clot. This is due in part to the lining of our veins being damaged, or there may be inflammation of the vein wall that can increase the risks of another episode of DVT.

In 1940, professor Keith Simpson identified the first case of DVT in World War II. He said that DVT causes fatal pulmonary embolisms to increase by 6 times in people who sat in air raid shelters for prolonged periods of time. In 1954 Dr. John Homans published evidence that DVT was associated with prolonged sitting during air travel. Since that time this theory has been believed to be true and has cause us to be conscious of getting up and moving around during long flights.

In a study at the Wellington hospital in New Zealand, professor Richard Beasley led a team of researchers that was studying seated immobility at work and the risk factor of DVT. The study showed that the longer the study subjects were seated, the risk of DVT increase significantly. The risk increased by 10% per hour longer seated at work without getting up. The maximum number of hours seated at work without getting up was associated with DVT, with the risk increasing by 20% per hour longer seated.

This means that many TV viewers, and individuals that are working in a sitting environment can suffer from DVT. This is especially problematic in some call centers, information technologogy centers, for truckers and other workers that have an opportunity to work more than eight hours per shift. Some individuals have the opportunity to work more days per week than five days per week, which really increases the risks of developing DVT.

According to Bacchus Vascular, a leader in the treatment of DVT, approximately 600,000 new cases of DVT are diagnosed each year in the United States. There are 20 million patients that have had prior DVT. Correspondent David Bloom died from DVT, from a pulmonary embolism in 2003. Up to 200,000 Americans die every year from pulmonary embolism, according to a white paper published by the American Public Health Association's Public Health Leadership Conference on Deep Vein Thrombosis (DVT).

DVT and the resulting pulmonary embolisms cause more deaths yearly, than breast cancer, highway fatalities & AIDS. Surprisingly, 74% of all adult Americans have little or no awareness of DVT, 57% were unable to name any of its common risk factors or pre-existing conditions that can lead to developing DVT. 95% of adults surveyed reported that their physicians or their employers or teachers had never discussed this medical condition with them. If we do not know about this problem it is impossible for us to be able to avoid the risk factors associated with this problem!

A recent study published in The Spine Journal looks at MRI changes in the discs in relationship to sitting. It is a very interesting study. The investigator looked at MRI scans at several points in time and looked at changes in the intervertebral disc in relationship to sitting behavior. They looked at MRI scans before sitting, after 15 minutes of relaxed sitting, immediately after seated unloading exercises and approximately 7 minutes after exercise," The authors reported:

After 15 minutes of sitting, mean seated height on stadiometry decreased by 6.9mm. After seated unloading exercises, the mean seated height increased by 5.7 mm. that meant that there was very little loss of height after the decompression exercises.

A few things are noteworthy in these reported findings. First, loss of height in the discs was apparent after sitting for only 15 minutes. Imagine what happens after sitting for

2 to 12 hour shifts in a call center or in an IT center! How about sitting and driving a truck on one of those 12 to 16 hour runs. What about when we sit for four to five hours playing video games or the five hours of sitting when we are in front of some computer & or television screen.

The most significant and important seat that we all have sat or we all must sit in is a seat in the <u>Classroom</u>! This is very significant because we will spend countless hours in that seat, normally 6 to 7 hours a day, five days per week. Students get infrequent unscheduled breaks during each class. To add to this long period of sitting is that normally we are instructed to be quiet, sit still in our seats and not to move around and disrupt the class period. Going to school is something that all Americans are required to do; we do not have a choice. These periods of uninterrupted sitting and immobility seems like an almost perfect breeding ground for present and future cases of DVT.

The research is very clear that our hearts, backs, waistlines, gluteus maximus, our legs and veins have been taking quite a beating from all of the sitting that we have been doing. Who would've thought that we could experience so much damage to our bodies that could manifest in many different devastating medical conditions and even death, from something as common as our seats?

To think that the lifestyle that we have created for ourselves, with all of the innovations and advances that we have made on our jobs, in our homes and in our recreation and leisure time choices. The things that we use to make things easier and less strenuous for ourselves have also become the things that are killing us. Most of us want to live what we consider the good life but it seems that the good life is really turning out to be bad for us. What can we do to turn this situation around? What can we do to fix this problem? What can we do to decrease our risk of having heart, back, butt, leg, DVT, P. E. attacks and obesity? What is the answer to this question? What is the cure for all these problems? It's the same thing that caused

<u>Them!</u>

Chapter 14

The Sitting Disease (Epidemic!)

The Cure: Sitacise!

The evidence and the research is clear and it shows that sitting for long uninterrupted periods of time is killing us and causing us to die sooner from heart attacks, DVT, PE and obesity. We are becoming overweight and obesed in record numbers as a matter of fact it is predicted by 2015 that 75% of all Americans will be overweight. We are exposing ourselves to back injuries and back pain as never before. Sciatica, ruptured discs, and herniated discs and compressed discs. Deep Vein Thrombosis, pulmonary embolisms blood clots, red and swollen legs that are painful to the touch. These are the results of sitting too long!

We have created a culture of couch potatoes that is prone toward breeding more couch potatoes. We have done it all in the name of progress. We have done it because we Americans are resourceful. We have done it because we Americans are inventive. We have done it because we Americans are innovative. And just as we Americans have done it we Americans will undo **It**.

Sitacise is an exercise program that we can do any place that there is a seat. Sitacise exercises have been performed in a classroom setting and the students were able to do the program as directed successfully. Sitacise exercises have been performed in a work setting without any interference with the regular performance of the workers duties. Sitacise exercises have been performed in recreational settings such as watching television and playing computer games without any interruption in viewing pleasure or game playing performance. Sitacise exercises have been performed while driving an automobile without any changes to the driver's driving performance or safety.

The exercises used in Sitacise program provides the mobility needed especially in the lower body, to prevent immobility and uninterrupted sitting for long periods of time. This is especially helpful in providing movement while on the job that is necessary in decreasing the risk of heart attack. Studies have shown that we have decreased the level of movement on the job and that this movement needs to be present to prevent the gene that causes heart attacks from causing us to have a heart attack.

The study also showed that it did not matter how much exercise is done away from the work environment, if we sit for long uninterrupted periods without doing any movement, the risk of having a heart attack increases. Regular, normal periods of exercise and sitting are totally unrelated. We can workout but we will be considered to be couch potatoes that workout without doing movements at work. Sitacise provides this movement and movement while we are sitting will keep us healthy and alive!

The exercises are structured to be done for a duration of 30 seconds every 6 minutes. The exercises incorporate leg and lower body movements that facilitates muscle contractions in the lower extremities that help keep the blood circulating in the lower extremities. Every time the calf muscle contracts it squeezes the veins within them and forces blood up to the heart. If the calf muscle did not contract for long periods of time the blood stagnates in the veins. This causes the ankles and feet to swell; this increases the chance of the blood forming clots. These clots can be broken off and carried in the bloodstream to the heart and then to the lung and cause a pulmonary embolism, which can cause sudden death! Foot & ankle swelling,wow!

Sitacise is conducive for preventing deep vein thrombosis, blood clots and pulmonary embolisms because the muscles are getting the necessary contractions needed to prevent blood stagnation and sluggish circulation in the lower limbs that can cause those conditions to manifest.

The duration of the exercises and frequency of exercises can be adjusted for as long as the participant that is doing those exercises wants to do them. This is only a suggested guideline that one can use. If this guideline is followed the participant receives almost 5 minutes of exercise per hour that will equal 40 minutes of exercise during a normal 8-hour work shift. But we can do as many or as few seconds and minutes as one wishes to do. Just be aware that your results will vary accordingly.

There are also upper body movements that when combined with the lower body movements, facilitates contraction of the muscles of the entire body. This will also provide a very effective way to replace the movements that we used to engage in before we had so many sit down jobs. We can exercise our whole body while we are performing our duties on the job by performing the exercises in the Sitacise program. As outlined in the example above if we do 30 seconds of exercise every 6 minutes, in 12 minutes we will have completed 1 minute of exercise. In an hour, 5 minutes of exercise and in 8 hours 40 minutes of exercise! Wow, We can work out while working and once our workday is over our workout will be over as well.

Dr. James Levine in his article for the Mayo Clinic wrote about Non-Exercise Activity Thermogenesis or Neat. To sum up the article NEAT is fat burning that happens when we do activities other then formal or structured exercise, such as a classic labor jobs, non-exercise that burns calories. Standing, generally moving around, and activities such as that.

The Mayo researchers theorize that because we don't do a lot of those things anymore that is why we are so overweight. They say that those activities used to account for an expenditure of about 1000 to 2400 calories extra per day. Just 350 adds up to nearly a whopping 37 pounds a year! Sitacise will provide that calorie burning activity that we used to have when we did those kinds of things on a more regular basis.

Because the Sitacise exercises are so user friendly and easy to do anyone with even limited mobility movement will be able to do them. If you're able to stand up and sit down, you will be able to do Sitacise. If you can use your arms you can do Sitacise. We can reclaim many of the lost none exercise activity thermogenesis calories by incorporating the Sitacise activities into our normal daily routine. If we do Sitacise we can successfully eliminate this obesity epidemic.

The next problem that we need to address is that of disc compression. As we saw earlier after just 15 minutes of sitting the MRI showed that discs were compressed by 6.9 mm. This is very problematic because most environments that we have to sit in, schools, offices, jobs, cars, truck drivers, buses, trains, policemen and firemen, require us to sit for longer periods than 15 minutes! This can cause nerve root pain, numbness and tingling, pain in the legs and feet and lower extremity weakness.

But all is not lost because there is a simple decompression technique that we can use that takes 10-20 seconds and will recapture 5.7 mm of the 6.9 mm that we lost when our spines were compressed.

1.Sit on the edge of your chair. 2. Push off the seat with your hands. 3. Bend forward and slightly round your back. 4. Relax the back muscles in this position for five seconds. 5. Then gently release the weight from the hands back onto the chair for three seconds. This takes about 10-20 seconds and it is time well spent to do it! Repeat every 10-15 minutes or as needed for relief.

We have provided you with some great information to help you have a healthy back! If you following the advice that we have provided for you it will make a lot of difference for your health. We recommend that you see your doctor and get his advice and approval before starting any physical program or following any of our advice.

We will now provide you with some general information to help you attain better physical fitness and overall good health. It is our goal to eliminate this obesity epidemic that is killing 1000 Americans daily! We also want Americans to know that they need to know just how dangerous their chairs are. Most people have very limited knowledge about the great risks attached sitting. With your help of buying this book for yourself & one or two for your loved ones and spreading the word about it, we

Americans can beat these problems. We are doing our part to save these lives and we know that you will do your part also! Tell everyone you can to join the movement and **just sit and get fit! Just Sit And Get Fit Now!**

Chapter 15

Sitting and Getting Fit!

I Just Want To Look Nice Again!

" I just want to look nice again, lose some weight, fit in my clothes, I don't have to look like a supermodel. I would just like to look decent, you know not so big."

If we had a quarter for every time that we heard those words we would probably be a millionaires by now. Many people are just desperate and say they just want to be a nice size again. They know that they cannot do the kind workouts that they see on some of those infomercials and they do not want to do those kinds of workouts and the good news is they don't have to.

Considering the new field of study, Inactivity Physiology, and the Nonexercise Activity Thermogenesis studies it is apparent that it is necessary for us to stop trying to reach our fitness goals by using the old antiquated programs that compartmentalize fitness and exercise into a structured program that is performed for a specific duration at a specified time. We are now becoming aware of the fact that we must incorporate movement and activity throughout our normal day during these non-specified movement times.

The non-exercise activity thermogenesis (NEAT) studies suggest that an individual can burn more calories and lose more weight if they focus more on movement and activity during non-specified exercise times. This is because even if a person works out for 3 hours per day very intensely there remains 21 more hours of the day that they could use to do normal movements and activities that would burn up additional and even more calories.

Just by doing activities and movements that would burn up an additional 350 calories per day, an individual could lose 3500 calories in 10 days. That a pound every 10 days, 3 pounds a month, 36 pounds a year! WOW. We will just start to waste away to nothing. How can we burn 350 or more calories per day?

We are glad you asked that because we know the answer. First don't get caught up in the hype that you have to kill yourself to do this because you don't. Secondly, do not make the mistake of believing that sweating is burning fat because it is not! We are just losing water weight in a lot of cases and not burning fat.

There have been many cases of wrestlers and boxers who have lost as much as 15 pounds in a couple of days when doing what they call *"Cutting Weight"* when getting ready for a weight in for a match or a fight. Once they have weighed in and made their weight, normally a day before the fight, they can eat and drink and they put back all that weight plus some. There was this baseball pitcher who said he lost up to 15 pounds on hot days pitching but within a few days would drink it back. <u>SO PLEASE DON'T GET CAUGHT UP IN TRYING TO LOSE MORE THEN 2-3 POUNDS PER WEEK! ANYMORE WILL BE WATER, NOT FAT!</u>

Sitacise has movements that will provide the (NEAT) activities so that we will be burning calories all day long instead of during those specific exercise times only. We can do this by following our routine of doing 30 seconds of our movements every 6 Minutes. This will help us burn calories all day long very easily. It has been estimated that we can burn 1000- 1500 calories per day using our Sitacise activity movements. In a week that is 10,500 calories or 3lbs (10,500/3500=3lb.).

Next we can find ways to eliminate unhealthy hidden fats from our diet. Just 150 extra calories per day turns into almost   1½ extra pounds per month. 18lbs.A Year. That what- A daily Flavored Coffee! A candy bar! If we just make these little changes we will find out that we can lose lots of weight easily. The little things can make a big difference.

Sometimes we think that it requires so much effort and hard work that we just give up and don't try. We must stop thinking that killing ourselves is the only way to get healthy and lose weight! Sure if we want to work out extremely hard and we love that kind of activity there is nothing wrong with that! Running a marathon, training for football, basketball, track, swimming, etc. we need to train hard and intense for those sports. But for just good health and weight control we can just SIT AND GET FIT!

But even for those who want to work out very intensely and take it to the extreme, if they have jobs that requires them to sit for long uninterrupted periods of time, they still have to make sure that they are getting activity and movement in to prevent the increased risks of heart attacks, deep vein thrombosis (DVT), blood clots and pulmonary embolisms (PE).

Sleep, most of us love to get it but few of us get the right amount or the right type of sleep. We must find out through trial and error what is the right amount of sleep for us as individuals. This can simply be done by getting different amounts of sleep on different nights and monitoring how we feel after each night of sleep. If we feel rested, alert and wake up on our own, without an alarm clock, we have gotten the right amount of sleep for us.

We may need as little as 5 or as much as 10 hours of sleep but we must find out what works best for us. Why is sleep important in relationship to weight loss? If we do not get enough sleep we will not have enough *"sleep energy"* and we will feel tired and hungry. We will also crave carbohydrates. We will try to get the energy that we needed from getting our rest from *food energy!*

And what do we do to satisfy our craving for carbohydrates and our need for energy? We get doughnuts, muffins, flavored coffees, energy drinks, candy bar, soda and a bunch of other substances that provide extra empty wasted calories that increased our waistlines and still leave us tired and unsatisfied.

That's why it's so important for us to get the right amount of sleep for us.

Also remember this that researchers are saying that the amount of hours that we sleep before midnight are almost twice as important in providing our bodies with much better rest as those that we get after midnight. Experts say that we should go to bed between 9 p.m. and midnight for optimum results. So let's try to get our rest so that we can lose weight and become our best! **Wow! Not only can we sit and get fit but also sleep and get** fit when we adopt the Sitacise philosophy! How much easier can it Be!   We Can Look Nice Again America! And We Can Do It A lot Easier than We Think! Join the Sit & Get Fit Movement Now & Start Sitting & Getting Fit Anywhere You Sit!

Chapter 16

Sitacise: Just Sit and Get Fit!

Just Chill Out!

"When I get upset or angry I go to the fridge and eat everything in sight. If I can get it in my mouth, I'm eating it!"

Emotional eating or stressed eating is a very common and frequent occurrence. When we are stressed we find ourselves in the middle of an eating binge much like an alcoholic on a drinking binge. And just as an alcoholic regrets what he has done when he examines the many bottles that surround him, we feel the same way when viewing the many empty food containers that surroundings us after our eating binge.

But is this all our faults, just a case of not having the will power to stop eating all that food? Let's examine this often indulged in phenomena to find out if that's all there is to this situation, or maybe if we dig a little deeper we can find out why we binge when we are stressed out or emotionally upset.

Having been involved in athletics and physical fitness for almost (43 yrs. Mark) & (35 yrs. Kathy) we have encountered many individuals who have told us that if not for the occasional binge eating, that they would be able to maintain their weight with relative ease. But it seems that there's always something that comes up in their and all of our lives that causes us to get stressed out and that's when we want to "PIG OUT!"

We begin to eat as if food is going to go out of style so we better eat all that we can before that happens. But why do we do it, why do we binge?

When we are stressed our bodies releases cortisol, a stress management hormone. Its job is to calm us down, but too much cortisol slows our metabolism and we don't break down the blood sugars and blood fats in our bodies as quickly. This is why even if we don't eat more food but the same amount while under stress we gain more weight. Next we begin to <u>**CRAVE FATTY, SALTY & SUGARY FOODS!**</u> Why couldn't we crave salads or fruits and vegetables? Life would be so much easier if we were stressed and we craved a big juicy apple. Why don't we?

The reason why an apple is the last thing we reach for is because we want comfort food! We want something that gets us fired up emotionally, something that satisfies us, and soothes our stressed out minds and comforts our bruised feelings. We are looking for a

"*<u>comfort food fix</u>*" and all of our drug of choice is going to be some salty french fries, a fat, greasy triple hamburger with three slices of cheese, a chocolate bar, some doughnuts, cream sticks, pizza, barbecue ribs, ice cream, we're getting hungry, how about you? We're looking for something to make us feel better! And this food does a great job of making us feel better. When the food reaches our stomach a message is sent to our hypothalamus, (it controls food intake) that we are calming down and to stop eating, this causes us to stop binging.

But that not the only thing that this food does. It makes us want it every time we feel stress out. Remember the cravings, and we do this every time we are stressed. And this happens all the time, just look at the news or read a paper or go to work or just live and you will see that there is a lot to be stressed about!

Stress also affects the way we store fat. Kathy was working at a stressful job in a call center. She gained 7-9 pounds during that time and most of it showed up as a gut that she never had before. She was our *"**guinea pig**"*, **No Pun Intended,** and I got her permission before writing that; I don't like sleeping on the couch! But this also reinforces the statement that we store fat in our abdomen when under stress. Abdominal fat or visceral fat is dangerous fat that can cause heart disease, strokes, diabetes and hypertension.

When the liver metabolizes visceral fat it is released into the bloodstream as (LDL) lipoprotein or bad cholesterol. This is the main culprit that builds up into the plaque that blocks our arteries. Visceral fat is harder to lose than subcutaneous fat that is just below the surface of our skin. It is important to incorporate movement and increased activity daily to get rid of it. Our Sitacise program will provide the consistent movement and activity necessary to accomplish this.

Stress can cause serious health related problems for us and there are many more, such as chronic job stress that causes burnout, psychosomatic problems, mental health problems, dissatisfaction with the job, ect. We have presented enough evidence to get our point across but what can we do to correct these problems without getting even more stressed out in the process?

The tendency is to ignore these problems and try to tough it out but these are serious problems that require serious and realistic solutions, not machismo messages of getting tough and working through it. To handle job stress try this technique: Sit down and slowly relax your body. Slowly inhaled through your nose and silently count to five. Let the air out through your mouth and count to 10 silently. Do that several times and relax. When you go on break find a quiet place for several minutes and sit down and become comfortable. Tense all the muscles in your face and close your eyes as tightly as possible and hold this for a count of 8 as you inhale. Now exhale through your mouth and relax completely just as you would when sleeping. Go down the rest of your body the same way relaxing these groups. The neck shoulders and arms, stomach and chest, buttocks, legs and feet, feel the tension come out of your whole body.

When we go on break we should not go for a smoke as a stress reliever. The chemicals in the cigarettes do not really relax us, as a matter of fact studies show that when we smoke we feel tense, anxious, stressed and on the edge. The carbon monoxide and the nicotine that's in the cigarettes reduce the amount and supply of oxygen to our brains. Without this oxygen we don't think clearly or concentrate very well. Nicotine is also a vaso-constrictor, it shrinks our veins and arteries making our heart pump harder, to pump the same amount of blood through the body. Our hearts beats 35,000 times more per day than a non-smoker and our blood pressure is 10 to 20 points higher than it should be.

Why are we so in love with something that makes our bodies respond like that? The nicotine activates reward pathways in the brain just as cocaine or amphetamines do. Dopamine levels, which are responsible for feelings of pleasure and well-being, are increased in the brain within 10 seconds of smoking. This makes a smoker feels good, real good, but the effects wear off within minutes. Now we start to feel irritable, anguished and stressed. So in order to get that good feeling again what do we have to do? We have to fire up another cigarette and we do this process over and over again. That's how we turn into a pack a day smoker!

That's why it's so important not to use cigarettes as a stress reliever, America. Think about how many poor, uninformed ex-smokers, or uninformed current smokers that think they are relieving stress when they take that break & smoke & all they're doing is increasing their health problems. Mark smoked for 25 years and he always says that it was an addiction that woke him up in the morning to get that 1st smoke and put him to bed at night to get that last one!

Please buy one of these books for someone you love so they can avoid wasting their precious years and endangering their health. Your lungs may start to repair from the damage of smoking in a fairly short period of time if you quit now!

Chapter 17

America Is Fat But We Will Cure That!

Why are Americans So Fat?

Last year Kathy & I came across a very disturbing headline:
it read that by 2015 75% of all Americans would be overweight! We began to research this headline a little deeper and found numerous studies that supported this claim. John Hopkins University researchers analyzed 20 public studies plus national surveys of weight and behavior and they concluded that 75% of all US adults would not just be overweight but obese which means more than 30 pounds above their normal weight.

Another report published in the Epidemiologic Reviews also forecast that 24% of children will be overweight by 2015. The obvious question that we asked each other was *"Why Are We Americans so Fat"?* We have access to the best fitness facilities in the world; we have some of the most renowned personal trainers and fitness experts in the world. Most important of all is that our government is bringing awareness and trying to find the answer to this question. This is what is known as the *"obesity epidemic,"* because it is so widespread and has reached epidemic proportions. It seems by the predictions that without intervention this problem is going to continue to get worse and worse.

So Kathy and I decided to embark upon a quest, upon a mission, upon a journey to engage in this *"battle of the bulge"* and to find out Why

We Americans Are so Fat! And the Great News Is That We Found The Answer! We Found the Cure for the Obesity Epidemic! We Know Why We Americans Are so Fat and We Know the Cure and We Are Going to Share It with All Of Our fellow Americans!

We are not going to let America becomes 75% overweight by 2015 or by any time! We Americans are better then that but most of all we Americans just need the knowledge to do better than that! Kathy and I have faith in all of us Americans! Now we are going to tell you why Americans are so fat.

Our journey began with us examining the two different groups of Americans that America primarily consists of. They are laborers and management or office workers.

During casual observation we noted that both groups as a whole were overweight, which is very interesting because one would think that the laborers having the harder jobs and having to expend more calories performing those jobs for an eight hour shift would be more likely to burn more calories, and be less likely to be overweight or obese.

So the first challenge was to secure, secret, employment in a physically challenging setting that required a lot of physical activity and movement that will require a large expenditure of calories. Once employed, observations would be made and questions asked to determine the behaviors and habits of the workers while at work and at home. We would observe & ask questions about food and drink that were being consumed at work & at home. Activities that were done other than work while on the job, (walking during lunch break ect.) and if any kinds of exercise was performed at home. Find out if workers went home and watched TV or were on the computer, or just sit around and rested most of the time when not working.

Mark was hired by a major food company as a labor and while employed there he made the following observations:

1.   There was a large population, approximately 60% 70% of the workers that were overweight. Most of the overweight workers seem as if they were not concerned about the extra weight or the risks attached to it. This attitude also could have been associated with feelings of apathy that many persons have when asked about a problem that is so personal, such as their weight. Some others had just given up and thought they were destined to be fat.

2.   Most of the workers showed little interest in participating in a structured physical fitness

program. A small group of workers had scheduled fitness matches weekly. Fitness DVD's & classes were offered but few wanted to participate.

Most workers that Mark talked to reported that they did not need to exercise because the jobs they were doing was exercise enough. The jobs that they performed were very physical in nature and some had to be performed in very challenging climates. This should have been more than enough physical activity to facilitate easy weight loss.

3.   Most workers had very erratic schedules and they had to check a list to find out what job & what time they would need to report to work the next day. This led to a lot of stress for many worker because of the uncertainty of being able to plan activities. Mark had many days where he

had to alter outside plans because of his job schedule. This schedule uncertainty could lead to increased job stress, which can be condusive to weight gain. It also made scheduling consistant workouts difficult.

4.   The workers that seemed to eat fairly balanced meals and drink normal foods. There was a need to decrease some of the fats, sugars and salts but with a little tweaking, their diets as a whole were not be too bad. When the amount of physical effort required to perform their jobs and the fact that most jobs required them to stand all the time while performing the job, these workers had to burn up lots of calories. So they could afford to consume lots of calories. During casual conversations, the information that they gave about their at home diet was consistent with their work diet.

5.   The workers seemed to go home and do some chores & then rest or recuperate from that days work. Some said that they went to recreational outings but most seemed to rest & relax. Summary: The workers work very physical jobs, the old saying "fat lazy Americans" is only partially true in their case Mark found no one in this pace that was lazy! <u>They worked very hard!</u> Management had a wellness-fitness plan in place but as with most of these plans they are more of a "you go down to the local club and we will pay half the fee & good luck to you! We'll put some posters on the wall; maybe have a well-ness committee of ex-jocks who used to workout & see what shakes out. But it takes more than that to help your most valuable resource; your workers get fit & most of all healthy! If you know the answer it's so simple to solve this obesity problem, but before we give it to you lets

look at the next group & see what office workers & laborers have in common that makes them both overweight & fat! We can't wait to find out how about you?

Chapter 18

Why Are We Fat?

Office Workers

We have already covered the problem with sitting for long uninterrupted periods of time in the preceding parts of the book. And we know that office workers and those who sit for long extended uninterrupted periods of time have many health risks associated with this.

But what do office workers, who sit on the job constantly and laborers who never sit on the job have in common that causes them to become overweight? One common denominator between both groups is the non-exercise activity thermogenesis. The office workers don't have enough movement in their day during working or leisure hours to burn enough calories for weight control. The laborers don't have enough movement away from the job to burn up enough calories for weight control.

Both groups do not expend enough energy during the day for weight control because they are missing out on a considerable amount of calorie burning that would be generated by them participating in more normal daily movements time or NEAT time. Both groups need to move more while they are seated and not just sit! That's why 60-70% of them are overweight; they just sit & don't get fit!

It is estimated that if we were to do movements and activities during the 15-16 waking hours that we have during the day. We could burn between 350 and 2400 additional calories per day and that's a lot of calories! If we burned up 350 more calories per day that adds up to nearly 37 pounds a year. When is the last time we lost 37 pounds? I didn't say when was the last time we wished we could have lost 37 pounds, but when is the last time that we did lose 37 pounds? IN ONE YEAR! WOW!

Wouldn't that be a tremendous thing to have happened to us? And to be able to do it without having to go down to a club or put on workout clothing or pay a monthly fee for a membership. To do it during the time of our normal day, during our normal routine, just adding a little movement, a little activity to those times. That really would be NEAT wouldn't it?

When we incorporate our Sitacise program, which does include the knowledge that one receives from the book, the new movements one learns from the poster & the new movements that are taught on the DVD's into our normal daily routine. We will replace the non-exercise activity thermogenesis that has been missing from our daily activities and movements since we became a society that sits for such long uninterrupted periods of time. We sit in the seats in a car, we sit in the chair at work then we sit in a chair in front of the TV or computer screen at home. That's a lot of sitting time that we can turn into getting fit time doing Sitacise! And we can do it in as little as doing 30 seconds of movements every 6 minutes! That's right 30 seconds of movements every 6 minutes and we can do these movements anywhere that we sit! Just sit and Get Fit! Just Sit And Get Fit!

The Sitacise program can be done by everyone and it needs to be because of all of the health risks that are associated with long uninterrupted periods of sitting. We need to adopt Sitacise, as the movements for America so that we Americans will not be 75% overweight and fat by 2015, but 75% of all Americans will

become healthy and fit by 2015! America Our
motto should become:

Just Sit and Get Fit!

Just Sit and get fit!

Just Sit and get fit!

Join the Movement!

Just Sit and get fit!

Join the Movement!

America just sit and get fit anyplace that we can sit!

We hope that this information that we have provided will be helpful to you and everyone else who has the opportunity to become exposed to it. We believe that office workers, school students, sales, insurance, call centers, collectors, truck drivers, fireman, policeman will greatly benefit from this information.

Sitting is something that we all must do so it is very important that we have the information necessary for us to enjoy it and do it in as safe and healthy a manner as is possible.

As we can see the back is an extremely sensitive and delicate area. We must have the knowledge to learn how to take care of it and let it take care of us. The information in this book will inform you to do just that but you must use it, you must apply it so that it can work for you. When you buy this book for yourself buy 2 for someone that you love like grandkids or grandparents.

This book should be bought for all call centers, IT centers, school systems, insurance companies, office heads, collection centers, sales forces, trucking companies, policeman, fireman and everyone that has employees who sit for long uninterrupted periods of time. This book should be required reading for all of those individuals so they can understand the risks they face when they are working in these types of jobs.

The information in this book will also be very useful for those who are in nursing homes or wheelchair-bound or have special needs. The illustrated movements chart and the DVD's will provide the necessary movement and activity needed to eliminate this obesity epidemic for our generation and all generations to come.

Get a physical before doing Sitacise movements. Please use caution when performing any movements and do not overdo it. It took us some time to get into this poor condition & health so it will take us some time to get out. Do the movements at your own risks and take breaks as necessary and do not overexert yourself!

A sensible diet of 30% protein, 30% heart healthy fats and 40% fruits & vegetables may aid in weight loss and help stop cravings. All claims by others contributors mentioned in this book are their sole responsibility and may not reflect the authors' view. The authors' reserve the right to edit or change this book as necessary or desired. The results you obtain are solely your own and there are no guarantees express or implied about any specific outcome. All rights are reserved and copyrighted laws prohibit any reproduction of any part of this book without the written consent of the authors. Sitting for long uninterrupted periods of time is hazardous to your health! If you have a job that requires you to do that; or if you are a student that sit for a long time, or you are a couch potato that sit for a long time, or you know someone that does, You Need This Book Now! Join the movement now to just sit and get fit and make anywhere that you sit a place to get fit NOW!

EXAMPLE: SITACISE MOVEMENT CHART

Sorry that this one is so small & blurry but if you go to www.sitacise.com you can order a full size one that contain 20 movements that you can

Do

ANYWHERE!

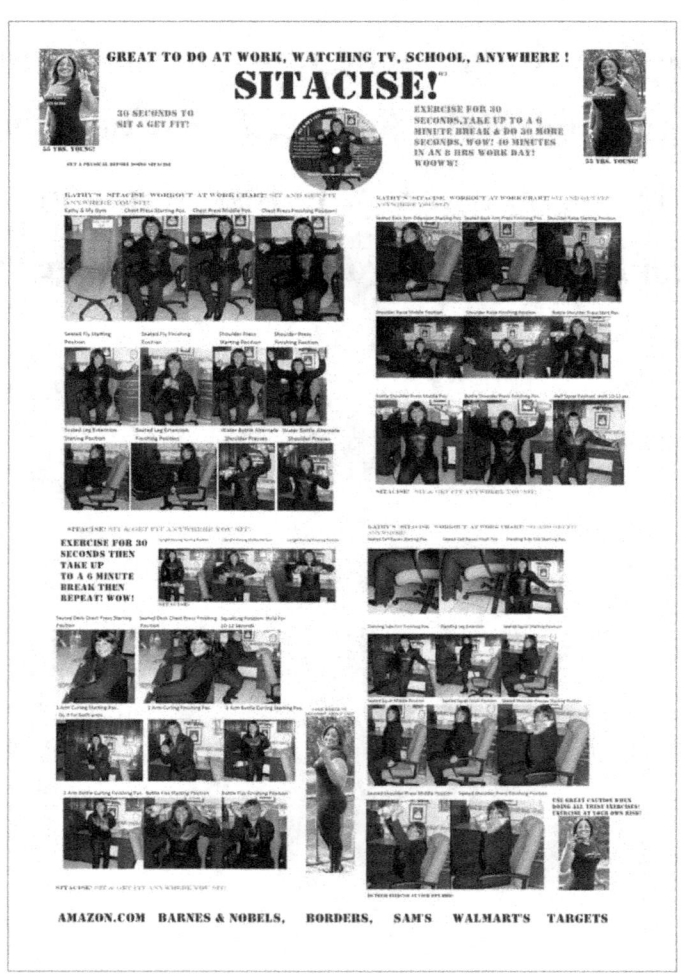

Bibliography

Wang, Youfa, Beydoun, May A. (Journal Epidemiologic Reviews,) 2007. 29:6-28.cEpub 2007 May 17

Nielson Media 'report "Americans using TV & internet Together 35% More Than A Year Ago" Nielsen Wire online_mobile/three-screen-report-q409/ 2010 March 22,

Anitea, Stefan,, "How does tv influence your life" news.softpedia.com/news/ 2007 December 14

Hersey Ph.d., James C., Jordon, Ph.d Amy "Reducing children's tv time to reduce the risks of childhood overweight: The media use study" Center for Disease Control & prevention Nutrition and physical activity communication team RTI project # 8680.006 2007 March

Hamilton, Marc, T., Healy, Genevieve N. Dunstan, David W., Zderic, Thedore W. Owen, Neville "Too little exercise and too much sitting: inactivity physiology and the need for new recommendations on sedentary behavior" Current Cardiovascular Risk Reports, 2 4: 292-298 journal article 2007-08 volume 2 issue 4 page 292-294 publisher Current medicine group llc 2009

Dunstan, Ph.d David, "Sedentary TV time may cut life short" American Heart Association Journal of the 2010 Jan 11

Journal of Applied Physiology, "Decrease in insulin sensitivity" Marc Hamilton reporting 2010, Oct 26

Levine, James, M.D., ph.d, "sitting disease" "NEAT"

www.mayoclinic/health 2007 Oct 26

Masters, Maria, "Why your desk job is slowly killing you" Mens Health 2010 10/26/

Katzmarzyk Peter, "Why your desk job is slowly killing you" Men's Health 2010 10/26 Hartman, Bill,

We want to thank all those who have contributed to this work through their past research which along with our present research will go on to benefit our fellow man and make a concerted effort to overcome this obesity epidemic, provide information about inactivity physiology and about the new sitting epidemic and the other dangers associated with it.

We will reveal the dangers associated with sitting for long and uninterrupted times to become common knowledge to everyone because sitting is an action that we must all perform daily.

Our research has contributed to further this exciting new field of study and we are looking forward to seeing what additional new information will be added to it. We want to advance the understanding of all our fellow men in this field as to facilitate the change necessary to improve the health & fitness of our society.

JUST SIT AND GET FIT IS THE EXCUSIVE PROPERTY OF
MR. MARK D. AND KATHLEEN M. BROWN, I. ALL
RIGHTS RESERVED AND MUST HAVE WRITTEN
PERMISSION FROM MR. MARK D. AND KATHLEEN M.
BROWN, I. TO REPODUCE ANY PART OF THIS BOOK.

FOR PROGRAM DEVELOPMENT OR SPEAKING
ENGAGEMENTS CONTACT THE BROWN'S AT
mbrown1 @ neo.rr.com FOR INFORMATION.

SITACISE! JUST SIT AND GET FIT ANYWHERE THAT
YOU CAN SIT!   JOIN THE MOVEMENT NOW!